Sex Art and Style

100 Sex Positions and Styles That Would Make Her Cum So Hard, & Scream Your Name!

TIM McCRAY

Limit of Liability

The information in this book is solely for informational purposes, not as a medical instruction to replace the advice of your physician or as a replacement for any treatment prescribed by your physician. The author and publisher do not take responsibility for any possible consequences from any treatment, procedure, exercise, dietary modification, action or application of medication which results from reading or following the information contained in this book.

If you are ill or suspect that you have a medical problem, we strongly encourage you to consult your medical, health, or other competent professional before adopting any of the suggestions in this book or drawing inferences from it.

This book and the author's opinions are solely for informational and educational purposes. The author specifically disclaims all responsibility for any liability, loss, or risk, personal or otherwise which is incurred as a consequence, directly or indirectly, of the use and application of any of the contents of this book.

ISBN-13: 978-1530087297

ISBN-10: 1530087295

DEDICATION

To all who desire to live life to the fullest!

TABLE OF CONTENT

INTRODUCTION

The art of sex and love making has evolved from the regular missionary position to more advanced and exotic sex positions that guarantees heighted sexual pleasure between couples and even more intense orgasms between couples…the women having multiple orgasms from their man's skillful touch. I'm tempted to say downloading this book might just be about the best buy lately, now don't mind me; I know you have gotten other good stuffs. This is one book that is founded by a great passion to see lovers to enjoy creative sex and explore new sex positions.

Many couples just oscillate between two sex positions and it's becoming something of a great worry. As they are getting tired of regular stuffs, and are fast becoming bored with how limited those few sex positions can be.

There's a great pleasure that comes from knowing what to do, and how to do it. Enjoy reading and have the best sex experience yet with your woman!

Ben Dover Sex Position

The woman needs to lean forward & balance with her hands, while the man holds his woman from behind. The woman needs a little flexibility and a bit of leg strength to perform this position well.

Both couple needs to face in the same direction while standing upright. The man then needs to enter the woman. When he has penetrated her, he then needs to lean over and stretch her arms out until she is touching the floor with them to balance herself. Ideally, she should try to keep her hands as close to her feet as possible, but if the woman is not that flexible or it feels uncomfortable, then you are free to lean forward a bit.

Basset Hound Sex Position

This position is a variation of the Doggy Style. It is named so because of the closeness of the couples to the floor. The position is straightforward; the woman is on all fours with the man holding on to the woman's bottom or the sides. Because of the low position the woman's rear is pushed right back, while the man's knees is placed to either side of the buttocks. The low position requires a degree of flexibility in the couple's hips and may not be comfortable for many couples but for those who can, the effort is really fun!

Bucking Bronco Sex Position

If you like being on top and having most of the control during sex then this sex position is great for you. The Bucking Bronco is very much like the Octopus position but is far easier and less exhausting to perform.

In this position, the man needs to lie down on his back. Then the woman needs to get on the top of him, facing him. When the man is inside the woman, she leans backwards and put her arms behind her to keep herself balanced. Then she puts her feet so that they are either side of the man's head. The wider she spreads her feet, the easier it will be to balance herself.

At this point, she will be able to bounce up and down on her man, just like a Bucking Bronco. She will find that it is quite easy to switch to the Bucking Bronco from the Reverse Cowgirl position.

Corner Cowgirl Sex Position

This sex position is a variation of the popular Cowgirl sex position, where the woman is on top of her man at the corner of the bed, while her man lies on his back. This is a position is fun to try out with your spouse.

The man has to lie on his back on the bed. His crotch is positioned by the corner of the bed, so that one of his legs dangles over one side of the bed, while the other leg dangles over the end of the bed. The man should plant his feet on the floor to give him some stability. The woman then needs to straddle him as she normally would when performing the cowgirl position so that she is on her knees, "bouncing" up and down on him.

Crab Sex Position

This sex position is a position that I will only recommend to couples in which the man has a good penile flexibility. The reason is because the woman will be bending his penis really far back when she sits on him.

The Crab Sex Position is in many ways very similar to the Cowgirl position, with the woman on her knees on top, facing her man while he lies on his back. Instead of the woman being in a semi upright position on top of her man, she will be leaning right back. She should make sure that she stretches her hands out behind her to support herself in this position. Her man should keep his legs together.

Fast Fuck Sex Position

As the name suggests this sex position is perfect when you want a quickie with your man. The Fast Fuck involves the man rapidly thrusting in and out. In many ways, the Fast Fuck is somehow similar to the woman on top position or even the Asian Cowgirl position.

The man lies down on his back and then he bends his knees slightly with his feet planted on the ground. The woman then straddles him. She has a choice of being on her knees or on her feet; the decision is up to her. But she will be leaning forward, resting on her hands or elbows. She needs to position herself so that she is slightly raised above her man.

Jugghead Sex Position

This position is likely the craziest looking sex making positions that you may see, even though to perform it is not as difficult.

 The couple is going to need to use either a couch or a bed to do the jugghead position. The man would need to set himself up first. The man lies down beside the bed/couch with his back on the floor.

The man then puts his legs up on the sofa or the bed. The woman then needs to position herself above him on all fours with one arm and one leg on the either side of him. The man now needs to lift his crotch and lower his back off the floor and then start penetrating the woman, while she thrusts back onto him.

Lunge Sex Position

This position's name originated from the way it is performed. The woman will be lunging on top of her man while performing it. This means that she needs to have some flexibility and strength if she wants to perform the Lunge for an extensive time with her man. Some folks see the Lunge as a novel sex position while some other folks see it as a regular sex position.

The man has to lie down on his back on the bed and he needs to open his legs. The women would then get into a lunging position on top of the man. She sets out to achieve this by standing up straight on the bed, facing the man with her feet together just below his crotch with her feet inside his legs.

Then she takes her left foot and then places it to the side of her man's right arm on the bed. Next she puts her right leg backwards behind herself so that she is in a lunging position and she lowers herself onto her man. With help from her man, she slowly lowers and raises herself on her man while he is inside her.

Missionary

This position is also known as the Male Dominant or the Matrimonial.

This is also the most used position in the world. It is an intimate position that allows face to face contact. The woman lies on the bed and the man lays on top of her, the woman could spread her legs wide open or she raise her knees and digs her feet in the mattress. The man likes it because he can control the depth of penetration and the speed of thrusting. She enjoys feeling the man's weight on her body, and the skin to skin contact. The only little downside of this position is that this position can make it more difficult to hold off ejaculation because of the intense friction and deep thrusting.

Rodeo sex

This sex position is a sex game of sorts, a sex game that you can only play once with a partner

Rodeo sex involves entering a girl from the back doggy style and reaching around and taking hold of her breasts. Once you are well inside of her, lean forward and whisper into her ear "I love you, Nichola" Or any other name that

ISN'T her's, or you could say "that's how your sister loves it too" or "that's how Sarah moans too"

The fun of the game now comes from seeing how long the man can hold on in her while she kicks trying to get you off.

Sybian Sex Position

This position got its name from the Sybian machine. It is a vibrator in a box that the woman straddles in a manner resembling the Cowgirl position, with a knee on either of the sides of it on the bed.

The Sybian sex position is similar to this idea above, but it has few differences. The first is that the man will be on either a bed of cushions or a soft cushioned stool or the seat. He will be lying on his butt.

This position can get very tiring, very quickly for the man. The woman will need something that her man can comfortably lie on that doesn't have any armrests that would inconvenient him.

The woman will still be straddling her man like in the Cowgirl position, except instead of resting on her knees on either side of her man, she will be on her feet, sitting in his lap while facing him. She can put her hands on her man or on either side of him to help keep herself balanced.

Thigh Tide Sex Position

This position is really fun and very easy to perform it. It's a great position to try out.

The man needs to lie on his back with his legs straight and also spread slightly apart. Now he raises one of knee slightly and then plants his foot on the bed. The woman now then puts one knee on either side of his bent leg and then he sit down on his crotch while facing away from him. The woman now uses her legs to raise herself up and down on the man. She makes sure to hold onto her man's leg to help steady herself. It is really great for slow and sensual sex!

Delight Sex Position

This sex position is a great for couples who want to be quite intimate. The position is also very nice because you don't have to put in that much effort to perform the Delight.

The woman needs to sit at either the edge of her bed or on a sofa or on the edge of any surface that is about twelve to twenty inches from the ground. When she is sitting down, she opens her legs wide. Her man then kneels in front of her, facing her. For the man to enter her, she may need to slightly lower herself over the edge. Her man will usually have his legs close together. He can then grab her waist or legs as he is thrusting into her.

High Chair Sex Position

This position is a fun position, a rear entry sex position, where the woman gets to sit and relax literally, while her man is the one who does most of the work. The only thing she will need to perform the position with her man is a tall stool or a bar stool

The woman is going to be sitting down on a tall stool or bar stool with her butt hanging out over the edge. So she is going to be sitting on the underside of her thighs, not her butt. The man will enter her from behind. Then she can now lean forwards away from her man or backwards into her man to find the right angle. If her man is not tall enough to penetrate her, then get your man to stand on something firm.

Don't put anything under the bar stool you are using, making sure it is on a firm, solid surface to prevent any accidents.

Ballerina Sex Position

This position is one of those super exotic ones that ninety five percent of women or ladies will just never be able to perform. This is simply because flexibility is key in this position. However if you get to performing it, then it can be very intimate and pleasurable.

The couple needs to start by facing each other while standing. The woman is now going to need to raise one of her legs upwards until she is resting it on her man's shoulder, while balancing on her other leg. Her leg that is resting on the man's shoulder is going to be almost straight, allowing the woman to be very close to her man.

Sofa Surprise Sex Position

This sex position sounds like the name. It can only be performed on a sofa, but it can also be performed when on an armchair, in bed or even on the floor. In many different ways it's very similar to the Asian Cowgirl

The man sits on a sofa as he would normally. The woman then squats down from a standing position on the sofa while she faces towards him so that he can penetrate her. She will be squatting quite far down, so she needs a little bit of flexibility otherwise it will be uncomfortable. If you are doing the Sofa Surprise on a bed, then the man will have to sit against the headboard and should put in a few pillows behind him for support.

Burning Man Sex Position

This position got the name from the fact that it is a passionate, fiery, 'burning' sex between the couples in this position. To do it, you will need either a counter top or table.

The woman needs to face the counter top and then lay her stomach over it while keeping her feet on the ground. The man can then penetrate her from behind either vaginally or anally. As her legs remain on the ground, they will act as an anchor, keeping her in place so that the man can really give her some hard, intense penetration without her slipping out of place.

Lap Dance

Get a tall-backed chair, pad the chair with some pillows, and sit the man down. Then straddle his hardened member and leaning back slightly, the woman placing her hands on the man's knees. Extending her legs, one at a time, until each of her ankles is resting on one of his corresponding shoulders. The woman pumps her booty back and forth at a speed that makes her moan. To super charge her thrusting power, balancing her weight between her ankles and her hands.

Pump Sex Position

In this position, the woman straddles a chair, with the man crouches on the chair seat behind her. The woman would stabilize the chair by holding its back, because care should be taken not to tip the chair and the man over in the excitement.

It is important to use a very good chair.

Slow Dance Sex Position

This sex position is a really fun position for the man and woman, where the couple is standing up. Well thankfully it's not as difficult as some other positions.

The couple needs to be standing while facing each other. If the man is taller than the woman, then the man needs to bend his knees and get a little lower than her so that he can enter her. To help the man to enter her, she will need to open her legs a bit. Then both of you just need to wrap your arms around each other and the man can thrust up into his woman. This position is great for slow intimate sex, while standing up.

If the woman is far smaller than the man, the Slow Dance will be impossible to perform unless she is standing on a stairs. But if she is taller than the man, then she can bend her knees and lower herself on the man.

Washing Machine Sex Position

This sex position actually needs a piece of equipment and that's a washing machine.

Find a washing machine, put few dirty clothes inside it and turn it on to a high spin setting. Then the woman needs to lean over the washing machine while still standing just like in the Burning Man Sex position. This will help to bring the woman's groin area in closer contact with the vibrating washing machine. The man will then enter her from m behind and start thrusting into her while standing.

Betty Rocker Sex Position

This position is one that most couples may never ever even come to trying. It may look a little out of this world, but it actually comes easy to perform.

The man needs to lie flat on the bed with his legs spread just a little bit apart. The woman then needs to straddle the man, but instead of facing him, she turns around, so that your man is now looking at your back. While upright, the woman slides his penis inside her, so that she is now in the Asian Cowgirl position with him. Once he is inside her, she starts to lean forwards slowly and rest part of her weight on her arms or his legs.

It is important to remember to start slowly in the Betty Rocker position so that she doesn't accidentally hurt her man!

Now the woman then starts rocking forwards and backwards on her arms and legs. But the fun doesn't stop there, the woman can also move herself up and down on her man's penis or he can thrust into her if rocking doesn't do it for her.

Bridge Sex Position

This position is a little stressful and you may be unable to last more than two minutes. It can be categorized among sexercise.

The woman needs to get into the 'crab' position that is used in gymnastics. The woman would be on all fours, except that her back will be facing the ground or the bed. The man now needs to get onto his knees between her legs while facing her. He then enters her and puts his hand on her thighs to help pull her towards him with each thrust. Keeping herself elevated in this position is very tiring.

Chair Riding Sex Position

This position is somehow exotic and takes two chairs to do it. If you do not use the right chairs for this position, you may find it to be quite uncomfortable.

This sex position takes fairly longer to set up than most other positions. First get two chairs so that they are facing each other, they should be near each other, so that they are almost touching each other. The man now needs to sit down on one and open his legs quite wide. The woman now needs to sit down on the other with her legs close together. The couple will both be facing each other for this position. Now the woman needs to slowly bring herself towards his penis while he brings his penis closer to her vagina. The woman will find that lifting her legs upwards will make it a whole lot easier. She may even find that putting her ankles over his shoulders like she would when performing the Octopus position makes it a lot more comfortable for her. Her man then holds onto her legs or grab her arms to gently thrust into her.

G-Spot Sniper Sex Position

The G-Spot Sniper position might look really unconventional but if you stick to it, you are and your man would really enjoy a great deal of experience.

The woman tries locking her feet together behind her man's neck to help her lift her lower body off the bed. The man then helps to keep her raised using his hands under her waist.

The woman needs to start off having sex with her man like she would in the Deep Impact sex position. This means that she needs to lie on her back while on the bed with her legs in the air, pointing at the ceiling. The man will be penetrating her while on his knees. But instead of spreading his knees apart to lower himself down towards his woman like in many other sex positions, the man needs to keep his knees together so that he is as tall as possible.

The man will then grab his woman by her legs or knees and pull her up towards him so that he can penetrate her. Almost all of the entire body will now be pointing towards the ceiling and the woman will carry all of her weight on her shoulders or upper back while holding onto her man's legs to steady herself.

The G Spot Sniper position is a little tasking, and it's not advisable to do this position if you have a bad back.

Jellyfish Sex Position

The Jellyfish is a little more difficult adaptation of the Kneeling Missionary. In this position, the man kneels up slightly while the woman sits into their lap, also facing him. The woman wraps their legs around the man; the couple wraps their arms around each other for support. This provides a better angle for penetration.

The couple together sets up a fluid rocking motion to gain movement during penetration - this resulting visually in a jelly fish kind of fluid movement, hence the name Jellyfish.

Life Raft Sex Position

This position may sound like a novel sex position for couples at first. But it's very pleasurable for several reasons.

The woman needs one of those inflatable pool mattresses that you can lie on. Some people call it 'lilos', some others call them inflatable pool beds. The woman needs to lie on her stomach on the mattress and in a pool, with her vagina in the middle of the mattress, while she is in the shallow water. The man then straddles her, with his feet on the bottom of the pool so that he is not sitting on the woman, pushing the woman downwards, but rather he is standing over the woman. He then enters her and starts to thrust.

Coital alignment technique (CAT)

This sex position a.k.a "grinding the corn", this sex position is primarily used as a variation of the regular missionary position and it is also structured to increase the chances of stimulating the clitoris during sexual intercourse (coitus). This can be achieved by combining the "riding high" variation of the missionary position with pressure-counterpressure movements performed by the couple in rhythm with coitus.

When this sex position is used as a variant of the missionary position, the man has to lie above the woman but he also moves upward along the body of the woman, until his erection begins to point down, and the dorsal side of the man's penis starts to press against the clitoris; and unlike in the regular missionary position, the man's body moves downward (relative to the woman's) during the inward stroke, and upward for the outward stroke. The woman may also wrap her legs around the man's. Sexual movement is focused around the pelvises, without leverage from the arms or legs. The rocking upward stroke (where the woman leads) and downward stroke (where the man leads) of sexual movement builds arousal that couple let develop and peak naturally.

Note the woman on top variant is known as the reverse coital alignment technique.

Little Dipper Sex Position

This position is a novel position that is more like a Sexercise than some great sex. This sex position is the sister version of the Big Dipper Sex position. This position requires strength to perform. But to save energy, the woman should rest down on her man's lap and let him do the thrusting.

The woman needs a sofa or a bed and a footstool or sturdy chair. The man lies down on the floor on his back in between the bed and footstool. The woman now positions herself over the man and sits down on his crotch. The woman need now places her feet on the footstool and her hands behind her on the bed. The woman is now going to lift herself up and down on her man using her arms like she would if she were in the gym and she was performing bench dips.

Octopus Sex Position

This position is one you may have never heard anything of. That's cool because it's a new thing to try between couples.

The man sits down on the floor and lean backwards slightly; the man uses his hands placed behind his back to support himself. He will find balance if his legs is spread. The man now bends his legs slightly. The woman now stands over him (each foot either side of his waist) and the woman now slowly lowers herself in a squatting position onto his penis. Once he is inside her, she sits on his lap and slowly starts to lean backwards. Placing her hands behind her back on the ground for support. Once she is leaning backwards, she then need to lift her right leg and rest it on her man's left shoulder. Now she lifts her left leg and rests it on his right shoulder.

Pearly Gates Sex Position

This is not one crazy position that requires lots of gym expertise or strength, though many couples are yet to try it.

The couple will both be facing in the same direction. The man lies on his back on the bed with his knees bent and his feet planted on the bed. The woman lies on top of her man, also on her back with her head above his and to the side while her man penetrates her. So the woman would look like she is Spooning while facing the ceiling. Staying balanced on the man is important, so the woman needs to spread out her legs and bend them so that she can keep her feet on the bed.

The woman should also spread out her arms too to stay balanced. The man can then wrap his arms around her waist or chest or under her arms, grabbing her shoulders.

Piledriver Sex Position

This position is quite an exotic position that requires a lot of time at the gym working on your flexibility. It can somehow awkward to do this position between couples, and once you are in it, it can be really uncomfortable for the couple. Both vaginal and anal sex is possible in this position.

The woman needs to lie on her back. Next she needs to lift her legs in the air. The man now needs to grab the back of her ankles and slowly push them towards her head. This will cause her lower back to start lifting up off the bed. Alternatively if it's comfortable, the man will keep pushing her ankles towards her head until all of her back is off the ground and the only thing that's left on the ground is her shoulders and the back of her head.

This will leave her very exposed (this can be a turn on for some couples). The man now needs to keep at least one of his hands on the woman's ankles so that he can hold her in place. To enter the woman, the man points his penis downwards which can be uncomfortable.

Piston Sex Position

This sex position will fire the couple up without tiring you out (not as compared to the other sexercise oriented positions) Reminiscent of Standing and Carrying, this position has the plus advantages of being very easy on the man's back who happens to be the lifter and more supportive for the woman who would be dangling in the air.

It's worthy of note to know that this position is quite challenging, requiring the standing partner which is the man to be fit and the woman, flexed and focused.

Other conventional sex positions that transits to this position are: Mastery (Suspended and Dancer). Despite our preference; for the man, the man should use proper lifting technique by always bending at the knees, properly keeping his back straight and coming out of the pose very carefully as he went into it ... for the woman, she should hold on as tight as possible and aim to maintain her balance close to her partner.

Sexy scissors sex position

The woman lies face up on a table top or desk with her hips perched on the very edge. She raises her legs to a ninety degree angle, and then the man grabs her ankles. He extends his arms out to his sides, and as the woman's legs are spread-eagle, he enters her while standing. And then, he starts alternately crossing and spreading the woman's legs like scissors, opening and closing as he thrusts into her.

Leg Glider Sex Position

The leg glider is one sex position that needs a lot of gym expertise from the woman, her flexibility should be a great deal, and her man doesn't need to be that flexible to do it.

The woman lies on one side, probably her left side. Meaning that her left leg, left side and left arm will be on the bed. Her right leg will be resting on top of her left leg and her right arm will be resting on her body, although she can put her right hand on the bed to steady herself if she wants. She needs to raise her right leg towards the ceiling while keeping her left leg on the bed. If she is flexible enough, her right leg should be pointing straight towards the ceiling.

Ideally the woman's right legs pointing to the ceiling should be at ninety degrees to the left leg pointing to the wall.

Mongolian Smurf Sex Position

This position is one very enjoyable position with the man on top, where the woman can relax and let her man do pretty much all of the work.

The woman needs to lie on her side in the recovery position just like she would for the Irish Spooning position. Then she raises her top leg a little bit towards her chest and puts her top arm either in front or behind her to stay in position. The woman can keep her lower leg fairly straight and feel free to position her lower arm how she like it. The man now straddles her straight leg while on his knees and remains upright and starts thrusting into the woman. The woman won't be able to do anything in this position so she can just relax and take it easy.

Poles Apart Sex Position

This position provides a lots of G-Spot stimulation without very deep penetration.

The couple lies on their sides, facing in the same direction. This looks like the Spoons position, but it's not. Instead of the woman lying with her head in front of her man's head, she needs to change her position so that her head is now in front of his feet and her feet are in front of his head. In simpler terms the woman should be laying head to toe with her man. The man then enters her from behind either anally or vaginally.

Screw Sex Position

This position is really easy to perform; it's a great one to try out between couples.

The woman starts off by lying on her side to perform the Screw position. Then once she is, she pulls her knees right up to her chest so her groin area is really exposed. The man will then be on his knees facing towards her and will start thrusting her. To get down to the woman's level, the man will need to spread his knees pretty far apart. If he can't, then the woman should try putting a pillow under her hip to raise herself up or the man can can kneel on the floor instead of the bed to get the angles right.

Side Entry Missionary Sex Position

Although it's called the Side Entry Missionary position, it's really doesn't look like the missionary position at all.

The woman lays on her side on the bed with her legs together and bent. Most women are flexible enough in this position to turn and face their man to increase the level of intimacy. Meanwhile the man will be on his knees and will enter the woman from behind. So the man will be in the same position he usually is when performing the missionary position, while the woman will be in a new position.

Sofa Spooning Sex Position

This position is a slight variation of the regular Spooning position. Performing it, a full length and comfortable sofa is needed. Sofa Spooning is good when you are on holidays and want to see movies on TV as you have sex.

The man lies down on the sofa with his back firmly against the backrest part of the sofa. Now the woman lies down in front of him while facing in the same direction. The man now enters her from behind and starts to slowly thrust into her while wrapping his arms around her.

Spoons sex position

This position is also known as spoons position or spooning is a sexual position that derived its name from the way that two spoons may be positioned side by side, with bowls aligned.

In the spoons position one partner lies on one side with knees bent while the other partner lies with his or her front pressed against their back. The spoons cuddling position isn't limited to twosomes.

In this position the woman would be in the inner spoon position and the man is in the outer spoon, preparing to penetrate from the rare. While thrusting, the couples can separate their upper bodies, with just their pelvises connecting; their legs can also rest on top of each other. The woman lifts her upper knee to allow for easier penetration. The man can also caress the woman's stomach and stimulate her breasts, the back of the neck and ears, and clitoris. The woman can also stimulate her own clitoris or the man's scrotum. In addition, the penis stimulates the front of the vagina, and may stimulate an area that is commonly termed the G-spot.

Spork Sex Position

This position is also known as the Spoon and fork Combo. The woman lies on her back, raising her right leg so the man can position himself between her legs at a ninety degree angle and enter her. The woman's legs will form the tines of a Spork, a Spoon-and-fork utensil. The woman can do this with him facing her or facing her back. If the woman is more flexible, she should lift her left leg up to increase the depth of penetration.

From the Spork position, she can lift her top leg and support it by resting it on his shoulder. From this point, she can easily stimulate her clitoris using her fingers while he is inside her.

Woman on top

The woman on top sex position is also known as the riding position or the cowgirl, it is a sex position in which the man sits or lies on his back, and his woman straddles her man with her facing either forward or backward, and her man penetrates the woman in the anus or the vagina.

Twister Sex Position

This position is a very exotic sex position, when you do it; it looks really out of this world. Well for the records just because a lovemaking position may be exotic, doesn't always mean that it is better. Also, just to be very clear, this position has nothing to do with the game called Twister.

The woman lies down on her side, probably her right side. The man will also be lying down on his right side, with his stomach facing the woman's stomach, but the woman will be laying head-to-toe with her man. This means that the head of the woman should be close to his feet. The couple needs to bend their left knees and raise them towards the ceiling. This will create a gap between his legs and the woman's leg.

The woman now leans forward and pushes her body through this gap so that her man's raised left leg is now above her waist, with the woman under it, but above his right leg. The woman will also be sandwiched between the man's legs with her left leg above his waist and right leg below. The man should now enter her and start thrusting.

If you think this looks complicated, you are very right, it is very complicated! It takes some practice before getting used to it.

Cross Sex Position

This position is different from the Scissors positions because the man lies at right angles to the woman. With the lower body of the man under both the woman's bent legs; the woman being laid back in the Missionary position. This angle decreases chances of skin contact but allows more unique penetration angle

Anvil Sex Position

This position is a variation of the missionary position. It's a very easy transition from the missionary position. Read careful before trying out as not to accidentally hurt.

The woman need lays on her back, like she would when in the missionary position. Just like when she is in the missionary position, the woman needs to spread her legs. But instead of her resting them on the bed, she needs to pull them close to her chest. The man then positions himself over the woman. But instead of resting on his elbows, he will be resting on his hands. With the help of her man, she positions her legs so that her calves/ankles are resting on his shoulders on either side of his neck.

Lap Dance Sex Position

This position has a lot of resemblance to the Back Seat Driver Sex position. This is a sex position where the man can really relax and 'enjoy the show' the same way he would almost not do anything in a strip club, though he has the option of being more active.

The man sits on a comfortable seat or sofa. He should sit far back in the sofa or seat and should also have his legs open wide. The woman will be on her feet and need to back up into her man. She needs to get a hold of his penis and guide it in to her vagina. Once he is in safely, she can choose to either grind slowly on her man while he stays deep inside of her OR she can choose to bounce up and bounce down on top of him with his penis deep inside OR the man can help his woman using his arms OR she can choose to lean forwards or backwards on her man, depending on how intimate the couple intends to make the lap dance sex position.

Bent Spoon Sex Position

This position is a variant of the Acrobat position; it is also one of the favorite positions for intimacy. Unlike its very related family, regular Rear Entry, the Bent Spoon offers incredible access to the woman's chest and neck while offering less penetration angle. To be in this position, the man lies on the bed with the woman lying on top in line with her, facing the same way and with knees bent. Since the woman doesn't have very much leverage, movement is mainly the man's responsibility.

Brute Sex Position

This position is a variation of the Reverse Amazon sex position, this time with the man on top; the Brute Sex position may be one of the tougher man-on-top positions. It is not the easiest position to do, but it does give the man a sense of control and power that is absent or low in most other positions.

To perform position, the man squats over the woman (facing away) while resting on the back of the woman's legs, which is brought towards their chest to expose them at a unique angle. If the man is comfortable with his balance, he can reach behind and under to give the woman some additional manual stimulation.

Butterfly Sex Position

The sex position is an advanced sexual position in which the woman lies on a low table, ottoman, or a bed and lifts her legs onto her partner's shoulders. The now supports her hips to allow for proper positioning.

The butterfly sex position is a really great position to do if the couples are looking for a way to liven up their sex life or they just want to try sex in a different location or room. They should ensure that the object they use is stable, and sturdy, and can handle some rough play. Enjoy.

Sliding Lady Sex Position

This position is like a reversal of the Coital Alignment Technique. Instead of the man being on the top of the woman, the woman I on top in this position.

Though this sex position looks a little awkward, but it can be incredibly pleasurable!

The man lies down on his back as if he was doing the Side Saddle positions or the Asian Cowgirl. The woman then needs to straddle the man as she would when doing the Cowgirl position. So she will be on her knees on top of her man, facing him. Then she needs to lean over him and rest her weight on her hands. This next one is the most crucial part:

She now needs to position herself so that her clitoris is in contact with her man's pubic bone. She does this by arching her back like a cat.

Reverse cowgirl

The man lies on his back and, while facing his feet the woman straddles him with her knees on either side of his hips. Or, if it's more comfortable, she should squat over him with her feet flat on the bed. When he's nice and hard (and of course when the woman's vagina is well lubricated), the woman places one hand on the bed or on his legs to steady herself, as she holds the base of his penis with her other hand, and slowly lower herself onto him.

Once he's securely inside of her, she starts moving up and down, using her leg muscles to build momentum. The woman can help maintain her balance by placing her hands in front of her (on his legs or the bed), or reach back and put her hands on his thighs. One of the major advantages of any girl-on-top position: the woman is in control, so she mixes things up and does whatever she feels best. She can vary the speed and depth of penetration. Or play with her movements by gyrating back and forth or in circles instead of just up and down. At some point, the woman should try arching her back, which allows his member to stimulate her G-spot. And, since the woman has easy access to her clitoris, she should give herself a hand if you need it.

Deck Chair Sex Position

In this position, the woman lays on her back, and pivots her hips so that her legs is in the air, and then she bends her knees while the man enters from a kneeling position while supporting some of his weight on the woman's legs. This position is a favorite of many men because of the sense of power that comes from folding their lover; this position doesn't leave the receiver out of the fun. When the man leans on the woman's legs, it better improves the angle of penetration to better target the g-spot, and increase satisfaction of the woman

Deep Impact Sex Position

This sex position is a variation of the Deep Stick sex position, but it is easier as the man kneels by the side of the bed or couch thereby lining up more easily with the woman. To get into position, the woman lies on her back with her legs resting on the shoulders of the man, who penetrates his woman from a kneeling position. This position also stays true to its name, meaning the man can thrust in with all intensity, unless of course he is too big. Any height difference or discomforts on the side of the man can be easily be fixed using pillows.

Downstroke Sex Positions

This position is also a variation of the Deep Stick sex position, but it is easier as the man crouches by the side of the bed, sofa or couch. So he lines up more easily with the woman. To get into this position, the woman will need to lie on her back with her legs resting on the shoulders of the man, the man then penetrates from a standing position. But due to the higher position of the man this variation is not as intimate as either the Deep Stick sex position or its other family the Deep Impact sex position.

Jockey Sex Position

This position got its name from the idea that your man would like a horse riding jockey when in this position.

The woman lies with her face downwards on her bed with her legs together and straight. The man now straddles her with his knees on either side of her waist. The man then enters the woman either anally or vaginally and starts to thrust. He doesn't have to lean forward as a jockey would do when riding a race horse but he can if he wanted. He can also lean backwards slightly in the Jockey position. The man can also lean right on top of her so that it feels more like you are spooning with him.

Drill Sex Position

In this position, the woman lies on her back and wraps her legs around her man who mounts her from above. Although it looks very similar to the Missionary position, the raised legs of the woman makes a significant improvement in the penetration angle as well as the intimacy, therefore making it a good first step for improving the sometimes monotonous starting position.

Exposed Eagle Sex Position

This position might just be one of the hardest positions to perform. It requires great flexibility and strength. If you don't have this gym or yoga expertise, then the couple is in for a pretty sore time!

The best way to get into this position is to start out in the Cowgirl position. This means that the woman needs to be on top of her man with her knees on either side of him. She then lies backwards until her back is resting on her man's thighs and knees while she is still on her knees. He can raise his knees if she isn't flexible enough so she is more upright. The man now needs to raise his upper body so that he is in a seated position. He can then put his arms behind him to support himself or he can put them around the woman's back.

Hang Loose Sex Position

This position is really an easy one to perform. It is a variation of the regular Missionary position. You don't have to sleep in the gym or be a work out expert to get into this position

The couple starts off in the regular Missionary position, instead of them lying with their heads by where the pillows are and their feet near the end of the bed, the couple lies across the bed. Lying across the bed will give both of them far less space. To overcome this, the woman should position herself so that her head and part of her shoulders are hanging over the edge of the bed. Her man will also be hanging over the bed, so he will need to extend his arms outwards and put his hands on the ground to support himself.

This sex position got its name from the fact that the couples are literally hanging over the edge of your bed.

Italian Hanger Sex Position

This sex position is great for hitting the woman's G-Spot while, and she also has a cool 'exposed' and slightly submissive feeling to it. It is very easy to make a transition from the missionary position into the Italian Hanger. The woman just needs to lie on her back

As the man is having the regular missionary sex, he would then need to get to his knees and bring them quite close to the woman, which will force her legs apart. When he is on his knees, he then needs to put his hands under the woman's bum and hips and lift them up. To help him out with raising her bum and hips, the woman bends her knees and plant her feet on the bed. This will allow her to push her waist or hips into the air.

The launch Pad sex position

It is one great way to get into a synchronistic sexual flow, whether the couple opts for deep and powerful thrusts or gentle rocking. It's also helps if couples want to achieve deep penetration and the massage of the woman's G-spot.

As in Deep Stick sex position, the woman lies on her back and raises her hips; the man now kneels down in front. Once the man penetrates the woman and begins to thrust, the woman's hips rise and fall in beautiful rhythm to every thrust. A positional aid can be placed underneath the buttocks of the woman, to help her maintain the elevation of her hips.

The woman's leg positions can be modified in many ways, like: bringing both legs over to a side, the man raising them over his shoulders, or keeping her feet together and spreading her knees wide. The woman can also place her feet on the chest of her man to bear some of his weight so that her man can lean over top of her legs; this gives a difference in sensation.

Missionary 180 Sex Position

This Sex Position is like a combination of two sex positions, the regular Missionary and the Betty Rocker Sex positions. For the man it will require quite a bit of flexibility in his penis to be able perform the position.

The woman starts by lying down on her back with her legs fairly spread out. The man will then lie down on top of her. But instead of the couples lying facing each other, the man will be lying head-to-toe with his legs spread out, resting on either side of you on the bed. The man now slowly and carefully pushes his penis downwards so that he can thrust into the woman's vagina. This will definitely put a lot of strain on the suspensory ligaments in the man's penis, hence the need for a reasonable level of flexibility, so he needs to be extra careful while doing this.

Pirate's Bounty Sex Position

In this sex position, the woman lies on her back with one of her legs resting on the man's shoulder; the other leg is wrapped around the man's thigh (the ship mast). The man penetrates her vagina from a kneeling position. Fairly easier to perform than its near cousin the Deep Stick, this position holds true to its name, meaning that the man can penetrate with every ounce of strength he has, unless of course he is too big. Any genital altitude difference should be corrected easily, by the use of pillows.

The Playing Of the Cello Sex Position

This position is a really enjoyable one for the woman. The reason it has the name is because the man will look almost like he is playing the cello with the woman's legs.

The woman lies on her back and raises her legs so that the legs are pointing towards the ceiling. Her man is then positioned upright, on his knees and penetrates the woman while facing her. The woman now rests both of her legs on just one of his shoulders, either the right or the left shoulder. The man now wraps one arm around the woman's feet and lower leg, while wrapping his other arm around her thighs, which makes the man look like he's playing the cello with his woman's legs, hence the name playing the Cello sex position.

Right Angle Sex Position

It is a really easy to perform sex position and doesn't require so much flexibility.

The woman starts by lying down on her back and pointing her feet towards the ceiling. She doesn't have to worry so much about keeping her legs perfectly straight. The man then sits down on the bed with his legs spread open. He should be facing his woman and sitting down on the bed just below her vagina with his legs in front of him on either side of the woman's body. The man now grabs her legs and lifts her up and towards him. He can then thrust into her.

The Right Angle got its name from the idea that the couple will be making a 90 degree angle, which is a right angle with your bodies in this sex position.

Sandwich Sex Position

This position is a little like the combination if two sex positions, the Viennese Oyster and Drill positions. It requires a little bit of flexibility and strength on the part of the woman.

The woman lies down on her back and let her man thrust into her as he would while in the Missionary position; on top. But instead of just resting her legs on the bed like she would in the missionary, she brings them towards herself while keeping them open. Her man's arms should usually be around her shoulders on the bed, but he would now have to lower them so that he can put one under each of her knees and help her to lift them upwards to change the angle that he's thrusting her from.

Tug of Love Sex Position

This position is one of a kind, and the last thing couples might actually dream of

The man first need to lie down on the bed on his back with his legs open. The woman then sits down on top of him and let him thrust into her vagina, with her legs on either side of him in front of her. Next She needs to start to lean backwards until she is lying down on the bed (she should put her arms behind her to ease herself down). Her head should be close to his feet. The woman can rest her legs on his chest or on either side of him, whichever is more comfortable.

Now that they are both lying down, the man should grab her hands so that he can pull her in towards him.

Victory Sex Position

The Victory is more or less the Missionary position but with the woman's legs extended out straight and forming into a v-shape toward the ceiling.

In this position, the woman simply lays down on her back while her partner lies face-down on top of her.

Viennese Oyster Sex Position

This sex position requires a great deal of flexibility. And most couples usually would get to a point where they can't continue due to the woman's inability to push past that point.

In this sex position the woman lays on her back with her lower back and legs raised all the way up so that her ankles are crossed behind her own head. The exact end position depends on the flexibility of the woman. This position totally exposes the groin of the woman to the man who lays on top the woman to penetrate. The man moves up and down on the woman to create friction. He needs to use his hands to support his own body weight so as not to crush his woman.

X Marks the Spot Sex Position

This sex position is really just a variation of the regular Missionary position. It's fun to try if the couple finds out that they are getting bored of Missionary and want something similar but more fun and different.

To perform it, the woman lays on her back while her man is on top. This position got its 'X' part from the fact that the bodies of the couples will form an X when viewed from above. So if the woman is lying down on her back with her feet at the end of the bed and her head at the top of the bed where the pillows usually are, her man will be lying across the bed, with his head by one side of the bed and his feet by the other side of the bed.

Bumper Cars Sex Position

This position is one very exotic position. To some couples this position is simple novel and to some others it is cool. Even the name is a little out of there.

The man must be sure to check that his penis is flexible enough. If he is standing up straight, then the man needs to be able to point his penis directly downwards towards the ground quite comfortably before even trying out this sex position.

If the man has enough flexibility, then you are good to go. Firstly the woman lies down on her stomach on the bed, with her legs straight and open wide. Then her man lies down on his stomach facing in completely the opposite direction and his legs straight and open wide as well. The man then reverses back towards the woman until his thighs are positioned over her thighs and he can pull his penis so that it's pointing towards her vagina. Then the man slowly needs penetrates the woman's vagina, making sure not to overstretch his penis.

Irish Garden Sex Position

The position is similar to the Betty Rocker position, very interesting and doesn't take a great deal of flexibility as it might look. It's very easy to perform.

The man sits down on the bed. He should have his back upright and straight, his legs out in front of him and also opened fairly wide. The man can bend his knees if he finds that more comfortable for him. The woman now gets down on all fours and reverses herself towards him. She will have to lower her waist down onto her man by straightening out her legs behind him (one on each side of his waist). Next she lowers her head and shoulders onto the bed until they are resting on it.

Doggie Style

This position also known as rear entry is a great position that has enjoyed popularity over the years, maybe because it comes with this naughty feeling.

In this position, the man enters the woman's vagina from behind as she is on all fours on the bed or couch. This position supports very deep penetration, as the woman's body is already being so angled; so the g-spot can be stimulated by each penetration of the man's penis. Depending on how far bent over the woman is and how fast the man can thrust into his woman. His testicles will also slap against his woman's vagina which can be really very exciting. Stimulation of the Clitoris is also very possible by both the partners.

Lotus Sex Position

This position is a popular woman on top position, it is also called lotus blossom.

The man sits on the bed or floor in the lotus position, his legs crossed or extended. After he gets into position, the woman now straddles his lap and wraps her legs around his waist as he pushes into her, wrapping her arms around his torso for support. The woman can rock back and forth in this position for more pleasure. The position also allows intimate touches and kisses.

Superwoman Sex Position

This position may sound like one of those positions where the woman literally needs to do alot of work to be the 'Superwoman'. Luckily for her this is not the case at all, the man does most of the work. In some ways the Superwoman position is quite like the Life Raft position.

The woman lies down on your bed on her belly, with her arms resting on the bed, stretched out in front of her. While her stomach should be on the bed, her waist will be at the edge with her legs hanging over the side. The man will then penetrate the woman while standing from behind and will start thrusting in and out.

Bulldog Sex Position

This position is similar in many ways to regular Doggy Style. However, this position puts the woman in an even more submissive position compare to the Doggy Style position. And makes you tighter for the man.

The woman gets down on all fours, on her hands and knees. Next she brings both of her legs together. The man then penetrates her from behind in a slight squatting position. He then places his feet outside of her legs and he can put his hands on the woman waist or her shoulders to steady himself.

Frog Leap Sex Position

In this position the woman squats, like a frog, in front of the man who kneels and penetrates from behind. The woman then arches her back to give easier access to the man, and the man should give a hand in supporting the weight of the woman as this position tends to lead to sore thighs for the woman in a short while.

Corner Doggy Style Sex Position

The sex position is a really great variation of the regular Doggy Style sex. While being performed on the corner of the bed or table, just like the similarly named Corner Cowgirl sex position, it has very little else in common with the position.

The woman starts off by standing upright on the floor with one of her legs positioned on either side of the corner of her bed or her table. The woman now leans over onto the bed or the table resting on either her elbows or her hands. Her man then enters her from behind, like he would during Bodyguard position or doggy Style position.

Bodyguard Sex Position

This position is a Spooning position with the fiery fire of the famous Doggy Style, the connectivity of a side by side position, and the erotic beauty that comes with the uniqueness of all standing positions.

The woman stands in front and is penetrated from behind by her man. This position is especially good in allowing the man access to touch and caress the woman's body. So make sure to keep those hands occupied!

The only difficulty with this position can be the alignment of the genitals which can be a real problem for some lovers.

It could be fixed by the following: standing on a foot stool, a stair, a couch cushion, or if the woman is up to it, maybe some high heels.

The Leapfrog Position

This position is also known as Froggy style. It is an interesting variation of doggy style sex position. In this position, the woman squats down but rather than getting into regular Doggy style sex position on all fours, the woman lowers her forearms to the ground and raises her butt so she can be penetrated entered by her man from behind. This position can be used for vaginal or anal sex. The man should support his woman's waist to help her weight. This position could take an extent of flexibility to perform.

Rear Admiral Sex Position

This position is great for those women that like to be dominated by their man. And in this position he is almost in complete control. The woman can perform this position while standing up or on her knees.

*while standing the couple faces in the same direction while both standing. The man now penetrates the woman from behind, either vaginally or anally. The woman now needs to bend over so that her stomach becomes parallel to the ground and she is facing the floor. The woman can spread her legs while the man keeps his own legs close together or vice-versa. Then the woman puts her arms parallel with her body. Her man then holds onto her hands or wrists and starts thrusting in and out.

In this position, your man can thrust in and out really hard and quite deep too if that's what you both enjoy.

*while on kneeling, the couples does everything as they would when they were standing, except that the couple will be on their knees. She spreads her knees wide and her man can keep his close together or vice/versa. The woman can also lean down a little and rest her head and shoulders on the bed if she likes.

That's the reason behind the name Rear Admiral. The man is in control of the 'ship' (the woman)

Stairway to Heaven

This position is also known as Step lively. This position is a variation on the Hot Seat with the woman sitting on top of her man while he sits on one of the stairs of a staircase! The Stairs offer very good seating possibilities and also a hand rail for lifting leverage and extra support.

Asian Cowgirl Sex Position

It is very similar to the regular cowgirl position. The woman stays on top; on the other hand the man lies down on his back. Though there are major differences that should be considered when performing it.

The woman has her knees either side of her man, resting on the bed in the regular cowgirl position. But when doing the Asian cowgirl with her man, the woman will be in a squatting position, which means that most of her weight is supported by her feet while she is squatting. She can use her hands to take some of her weight by putting them on either her man's chest or on either side of him on the bed. If she is not very strong or flexible, she will find the Asian cowgirl position to be exhaustive.

Fire Hydrant Sex Position

This position is a variant of the regular Doggy Style that some couples love while others are not so into it. To get into this position simply requires a little bit of flexibility.

The couple needs to get into the regular Doggy Style position. This means that the woman gets down on all fours, facing towards the floor. The man will then be on his knees behind her. He has to have his knees inside the woman's. The man is then going to have to start lifting one of his legs upwards and forwards and planting his foot on the floor to his woman's side. In so doing he will raise her leg on that side, so that her thigh will now be resting on top the man's thigh. This will make the woman look like a dog peeing on a fire hydrant.

Turtle Sex Position

This position is a type of Doggy Style sex position that requires a little bit of flexibility. It's a nice way to rev the excitement engines up when u start getting bored of the regular Doggy Style.

The woman rests with her knees on the floor. When in she's in this position, she lowers herself downwards so that her bum is sitting on top of the back of her ankles. Next she leans as far forward as she can possibly lean. She can grab hold of her legs in the front of her to help her lean further forward. Her man will be on his knees behind her thrusting into her. The man may find that he needs to adjust his height to make it easier for himself by either spreading his knees or bringing them together.

Bended Knee Sex Position

This position is a variation on the Dancer position; it is also a lot of fun if the couple is looking for something with face-to-face more intimate contact. The couples simply kneel facing each other. The woman simply raises one of her legs over the man's opposite thigh to give easier access while the man helps support her.

Book Ends Sex Position

This position comes really interesting. A lot of couples that wants to perform it may actually find it very difficult to penetrate comfortably. That's not to say that it's not a fun love making position though!

The couple would be on their knees facing each other on their bed. The man spreads out his knees so that he can lower himself while the woman will need to remain as tall as possible. When the man is then a little below her, he can now slide in his penis (the woman can be of helping, guiding in his penis). If it's comfortable, the man can then bring his legs together again and start to raise himself upwards. The woman can also lean backwards to make penetration deeper and more enjoyable for the man.

If the man is much taller than the woman, then she probably won't be able to perform actual penetrative sex in this sex position

Dublin Shuffle Sex Position

This position is one characterized with great fun and is great for lovers who value the intimacy of facing each other during sex along with the fun of both being upright while doing it. The reason it is called the Dublin Shuffle is because there is often a lot of shuffling when trying to find the exact right angle or 'spot'.

The man starts by standing on the floor, while the woman kneels on the bed. The couple will face each other. Before the couple goes any further, it is important to make certain that the base of his penis is at about the same height as her vagina. If not, the couple should put a few sturdy books under the bed to raise it, or the man should stand on something so that both the couples are at the right height. When the couple is both at a good height, the man can then penetrate her.

Shoe Shiner Sex Position

This position has a little bit in common with the Bended Knee Sex position as both the couple is facing each other while on just one knee.

The couple would face each other on their knees. They should be so close that they would be hugging each other.

They are both going to raise their left knees so that their thighs are parallel to the bed and their lower legs are vertical with their left feet firmly on the bed. This will allow the man to penetrate her easily. If the man is a lot taller than the woman in this position, then the woman needs to put a pillow or a cushion under her knee to raise her high enough.

Teaspooning Sex Position

Teaspooning sex position is a variation of the regular Spooning position, and might actually be one of the most intimate sex positions of all time. It is also very easy to move from doggy-style position to this position.

The man gets to his knees on either the bed or the floor. He needs to open his knees fairly wide. The woman now gets on her knees also while facing in the same direction as her man in front of him.

The woman should have her knees together so that her man can come up close behind her and penetrate her. When he does, the man should wrap his arms around the woman. He can put them around her waist or on her breasts or under her arms to hold onto her shoulders.

After Dinner Sex Position

This position is somehow similar to the Back Seat Driver position. The name comes from the fact that you use a table and chair to perform it, making it perfect for right after dinner or after a meal.

The man needs to sit on a chair that is two feet from a table facing it, while his legs are open quite wide. The woman now needs to back herself up into her man with her legs quite close together in a standing position. Optionally, her man can then lift his legs up from the ground and place them on the table. Once he does this, the woman will be 'trapped' between his legs.

The Back Seat Driver Sex Position

When having sex in this position, the man will sit on the edge of a sofa, a chair or even the bed with the man's legs spread wide and his feet on the floor. The woman now backs up onto your man's crotch and let him slowly thrust into her while bending her knees.

When the man is comfortably inside her, she will use her legs to bounce up and down on him. The couple will be facing in the same direction for this position.

Twister Sex Position

This position is a very exotic sex position, when you do it; it looks really out of this world. Well for the records just because a lovemaking position may be exotic, doesn't always mean that it is better. Also, just to be very clear, this position has nothing to do with the game called Twister.

The woman lies down on her side, probably her right side. The man will also be lying down on his right side, with his stomach facing the woman's stomach, but the woman will be laying head-to-toe with her man. This means that the head of the woman should be close to his feet. The couple needs to bend their left knees and raise them towards the ceiling. This will create a gap between his legs and the woman's leg.

The woman now leans forward and pushes her body through this gap so that her man's raised left leg is now above her waist, with the woman under it, but above his right leg. The woman will also be sandwiched between the man's legs with her left leg above his waist and right leg below. The man should now enter her and start thrusting.

If you think this looks complicated, you are very right, it is very complicated! It takes some practice before getting used to it.

Bouncing Spoon Sex Position

This position is a sort of pseudo-spooning position for couples. It is fairly easy to perform and a good option to liven up sex in the bedroom.

The man sits upright in bed with his back to the wall and his legs together and fairly straight (it doesn't have to be perfectly straight). The woman now needs to stand right over him with her back to him. Her feet should be on either side of his thighs. She then need to get down on her knees from this position and sit back onto the man's crotch and guide his penis inside her. She can now lean backwards so that her back is on her man's chest.

Lotus Sex Position

This position is a popular woman on top position, it is also called lotus blossom.

The man sits on the bed or floor in the lotus position, his legs crossed or extended. After he gets into position, the woman now straddles his lap and wraps her legs around his waist as he pushes into her, wrapping her arms around his torso for support. The woman can rock back and forth in this position for more pleasure. The position also allows intimate touches and kisses.

Mastery Sex Position

This is a great position that encourages intimacy, as it is very well face to face. That's good news for those that like a lot of kissing during sex. In this position the woman sits on man facing him. This position isn't great for generating vertical movement, so if you want to experience the full effect, it is important to try it on a stool or chair that lets the woman get a good footing.

See Saw Sex Position

This position is a really fun one, but couples get tired easily. There are really no similar positions to it, making it quite special. It also makes a good change from Doggy Style position or regular Missionary position.

The man sits on the bed. The woman then sits on his lap while facing her man. Next the woman should spread her legs out wide so that she is comfortable. She then needs to lean backwards and put her arms either on his shoulders or behind her. This position allows her to either move up and down on his penis or grind forwards and backwards on him all while facing her man.

Side Ride Sex Position

This position is basically a variation of the regular Asian Cowgirl position. It is very easy to perform and is good if the woman wants to be on top of her man during sex.

The man needs to lie down on his back like he would during the Cowgirl position. He would bend his knees slightly so that he can put his feet on the bed to give him some leverage for penetration. The woman now sits on her man's lap, allowing him to penetrate her. But instead of facing him or having her back to him, she is going to be sitting sideways on him. This means that she can sit on him with her feet on either the left side or the right side of him.

Side Saddle Sex Position

This position is superb for when the woman wants to be dominant and she just wants her man to relax and take it easy during sex. It's a great position to transfer to after blow-jobbing your man

The man lies down on his back on the bed. The man would have his butt at the edge of the bed with his legs hanging over it with his feet on the floor. He chooses how he positions his legs. Either together or spread out. The woman stands over her man with her back to him. She can sit down on top of him while spreading her legs if his legs are closed and together. But if he has his legs open then she would need to sit on top of him with her legs closed and together.

Final Furlong Sex Position

This position is a rear entry position that is physically very intimate. It is characterized by an ingenious use of an ottoman. It is similar to the teaspoon sex position.

71

The couples can replicate the sex position by hopping assuming the same stance a jockey would usually take in a race, by first mounting the 'saddle' (if the couple doesn't have an ottoman, a low couch arm can be used). The rear jockey which is the woman pulls the man in close and begins rocking his hips forward and back.

To create more movement and better penetration, the woman can raise herself off the ottoman slightly by simply putting more weight on her feet or leaning further forward. Be rest assured, there will be enough momentum gathered by the forward and backward motion to satisfy the woman's needs.

Carnal Crisscross

The woman starts by lying on her side with her arms above her head. The man on his side and his body perpendicular to the woman's, the woman slowly raises her top leg and let him inch his lower body between her legs. Once the couple is joined at the groin, the man should grab her shoulders while she anchors herself on the floor. The couple will need to hold on tight for this stellar trip!

END

Thank you for reading my book. If you enjoyed it, won't you please take a moment to look at my other titles?

Thanks!

Tim McCray